A Guide to Hysterectomy:

Empowering Your Journey to Health and Healing

By

Dr. Rachel Stratford

Copyright@2023 Dr Rachel Stratford

TABLE OF CONTENTS

Introduction

Welcome to the "Hysterectomy Cookbook," a culinary guide designed specifically for individuals who have undergone a hysterectomy. This cookbook aims to provide delicious and nutritious recipes that support your recovery and overall well-being.

A hysterectomy is a significant surgical procedure that involves the removal of the uterus. While it can bring relief from various health conditions, it also requires special attention to nutrition and self-care during the recovery process. This cookbook is here to help you navigate this journey by offering a wide range of recipes tailored to your specific needs.

Whether you are looking for comforting soups, nourishing smoothies, or satisfying main courses, "A Guide to Hysterectomy" has got you covered. Each recipe includes detailed instructions, nutritional information, and tips for adapting them to your dietary preferences or restrictions.

Additionally, we have included a section on post-hysterectomy self-care, providing guidance on managing common symptoms, promoting physical activity, and maintaining emotional well-being. We believe that a holistic approach to recovery is essential, and this cookbook aims to support you in every aspect of your healing journey.

We hope that "A Guide to Hysterectomy" becomes a trusted companion in your kitchen, offering not only nourishment but also inspiration and comfort. Remember, taking care of yourself is a priority, and this cookbook is here to make that process a little easier and more enjoyable.

Happy cooking and happy healing!

Chapter 1

Preparing for Your Hysterectomy

A hysterectomy is a surgical procedure in which the uterus is removed. It can be done for various reasons, such as treating certain medical conditions like uterine fibroids, endometriosis, or certain types of cancer. The impact of a hysterectomy on diet can vary depending on the individual and the specific circumstances of the surgery.

In general, after a hysterectomy, it is important to focus on maintaining a healthy and balanced diet to support overall well-being and recovery. Here are a few things to consider:

1. Adequate nutrition: It is important to consume a variety of nutrient-rich foods to support healing and recovery. This includes eating a balanced diet that includes fruits, vegetables, whole grains, lean proteins, and healthy fats.

2. Fiber intake: Some women may experience changes in bowel movements after a hysterectomy. Consuming an adequate amount of fiber can help prevent constipation. Good sources of fiber include whole grains, fruits, vegetables, and legumes.

3. Fluid intake: Staying hydrated is important for overall health and can also help prevent

constipation. Aim to drink plenty of water throughout the day.

4. Iron-rich foods: If the hysterectomy involved removal of the ovaries, there may be a decrease in estrogen levels, which can lead to a higher risk of developing iron deficiency anemia. Including iron-rich foods in your diet, such as lean meats, beans, fortified cereals, and leafy green vegetables, can help maintain adequate iron levels.

5. Hormonal changes: Depending on the type of hysterectomy, there may be hormonal changes that can affect metabolism and weight management.

Preparing for Surgery and Nutrition: Lifestyle Recommendations.

When it comes to preparing for surgery, Proper nutrition and lifestyle choices play a vital role in your hysterectomy journey. Here are some key recommendations:

1. Balanced Diet: Focus on consuming a well-balanced diet that includes a variety of fruits, vegetables, whole grains, lean proteins, and healthy fats. This can help provide your body with the necessary nutrients for healing and recovery.

2. Adequate Protein Intake: Protein is essential for tissue repair and wound healing. Include sources of lean protein such as chicken, fish, tofu, beans, and lentils in your meals.

3. Hydration: Stay well-hydrated by drinking plenty of water throughout the day. Proper hydration can help with digestion, circulation, and overall well-being.

4. Fiber-Rich Foods: Include fiber-rich foods like whole grains, fruits, vegetables, and legumes in your diet to promote regular bowel movements and prevent constipation, which can be common after surgery.

5. Limit Processed Foods: Try to minimize your intake of processed foods, sugary snacks, and beverages, as they may hinder the healing process and contribute to inflammation.

6. Avoid Alcohol and Smoking: It's important to avoid alcohol and smoking before and after surgery, as they can interfere with the healing process and increase the risk of complications.

7. Physical Activity: Engage in light physical activity as recommended by your doctor. Gentle exercises like walking can help improve circulation and promote healing.

8. Stress Management: Prioritize stress management techniques such as deep breathing exercises, meditation, or engaging in activities that help you relax and unwind.

Post-Surgery Recovery Diet: Nourishing Your Body

Post-surgery recovery diet is an important aspect of healing after a hysterectomy. It involves consuming foods that are nourishing and promote healing.

1. Adequate Protein Intake: Protein is essential for tissue repair and recovery. Include lean meats, poultry, fish, eggs, dairy products, legumes, and

plant-based protein sources like tofu and tempeh in your diet.

2. Nutrient-Dense Foods: Focus on consuming a variety of fruits, vegetables, whole grains, and healthy fats. These foods provide essential vitamins, minerals, and antioxidants that support healing and boost your immune system.

3. Hydration: Staying hydrated is crucial for recovery. Drink plenty of water throughout the day and limit caffeinated and sugary beverages.

4. Fiber-Rich Foods: Constipation is a common issue after surgery. Include high-fiber foods like

whole grains, fruits, vegetables, and legumes to promote regular bowel movements.

5. Omega-3 Fatty Acids: These healthy fats have anti-inflammatory properties and can aid in the healing process. Include fatty fish like salmon, walnuts, chia seeds, and flaxseeds in your diet.

6. Avoid Processed Foods: Minimize the consumption of processed foods, as they are often high in unhealthy fats, sodium, and added sugars. These can hinder the healing process and increase inflammation.

CHAPTER 2

Easy and Nutritious Recipes for the Healing Phase

After undergoing a hysterectomy, nourishing your body with the right foods is crucial for a smooth recovery. This presents a collection of gentle, easy-to-prepare recipes designed to support your healing journey.

1. Soft and Pureed Foods:

- Mashed sweet potatoes with a touch of cinnamon and nutmeg

- Creamy cauliflower mash

- Pureed vegetable soups (carrot, butternut squash, or broccoli)

- Smooth and creamy hummus with soft pita

bread or crackers

- Avocado and banana smoothie

2. Soups and Broths:

- Chicken noodle soup with tender chicken and

soft noodles

- Lentil soup with vegetables and herbs

- Creamy tomato soup with a side of grilled

cheese sandwich

- Vegetable broth with soft-cooked vegetables

- Creamy mushroom soup with a sprinkle of fresh herbs

3. Smoothies and Shakes:

- Berry and yogurt smoothie with a scoop of

protein powder

- Green smoothie with spinach, banana, and almond milk

- Peanut butter and banana shake with a dash of honey

- Mango and coconut milk smoothie

- Chocolate protein shake with almond milk and a handful of spinach

These recipes can provide the necessary nutrients, be easy to digest, and help in the healing process.

Cooking Tips and Techniques for Hysterectomy Patients

"Navigating the kitchen after a hysterectomy can feel like a new adventure. With a few smart techniques, you can make this transition seamless. Opt for easy-to-prep, nutrient-packed ingredients. Embrace batch cooking for convenience without compromising on nutrition. Experiment with gentle spices and herbs to add flavor without overwhelming sensitive palates. Don't forget the power of hydration; infuse water with fruits and herbs for a refreshing twist. Above all, listen to your body - it knows what it needs. Cooking for recovery can be a therapeutic journey in itself, and these tips will help you savor it."

1. Focus on Nutrient-Rich Foods: Encourage the use of nutrient-dense ingredients such as fruits, vegetables, whole grains, lean proteins, and healthy fats. These foods can help with healing and provide essential nutrients.

2. Incorporate Anti-Inflammatory Ingredients: Include ingredients with anti-inflammatory properties, such as turmeric, ginger, garlic, and leafy greens. These can help reduce inflammation and promote healing.

3. Emphasize Fiber-Rich Foods: Encourage the consumption of high-fiber foods like whole grains, legumes, fruits, and vegetables. Fiber can

help prevent constipation, which is a common issue after surgery.

4. Promote Hydration: Remind readers to stay hydrated by drinking enough water throughout the day. Hydration is important for overall health and can aid in digestion.

5. Encourage Small, Frequent Meals: Suggest eating smaller, more frequent meals rather than large meals. This can help prevent discomfort and aid in digestion.

6. Provide Easy-to-Follow Recipes: Include simple and easy-to-follow recipes that are nutritious and easy to prepare. Consider including

recipes that are gentle on the digestive system, such as soups, stews, and steamed vegetables.

7. Offer Substitution Options: Provide alternative ingredient options for those with dietary restrictions or preferences. For example, suggest plant-based protein sources for those who prefer a vegetarian or vegan diet.

8. Discuss Cooking Techniques: Explain cooking techniques that can help retain nutrients in the food, such as steaming, baking, and sauteing with minimal oil. Avoid deep-frying or heavily processed foods.

Gradual Transition to Regular Foods: Reintroducing Solid Foods

 it's important to note that every individual's experience may vary. After a hysterectomy, transitioning from soft and liquid foods back to a regular diet is an important step in your recovery. This will guide you through the process of reintroducing solid foods in a gentle and gradual manner.

That being said, a gradual transition to regular foods is typically recommended after any surgery, including a hysterectomy. Here are a few general tips:

1. Start with soft and easily digestible foods: In the initial stages, it's common to begin with foods that are easy on the digestive system. This may include foods like soups, broths, pureed vegetables, mashed potatoes, and yogurt.

2. Introduce a variety of foods gradually: As your body adjusts and heals, you can slowly introduce a wider range of foods. This may include cooked vegetables, lean proteins (such as chicken or fish), whole grains, and fruits.

3. Listen to your body: Pay attention to how your body reacts to different foods. If you experience any discomfort or digestive issues, it may be a

sign to adjust your diet or avoid certain foods temporarily.

4. Stay hydrated: Drinking enough water is important for overall health and recovery. Make sure to stay hydrated throughout the day.

Healthy Meal Planning: Balancing Nutrients and Supporting Healing

When it comes to meal planning, it's important to focus on incorporating a variety of nutrient-dense foods into your diet. This includes fruits, vegetables, whole grains, lean proteins, and healthy fats. These foods provide essential vitamins, minerals, and antioxidants that support overall health and healing.

To balance nutrients in your meals, you can follow these general guidelines:

1. Include a variety of colorful fruits and vegetables in your meals. These provide essential vitamins, minerals, and fiber.

2. Choose whole grains like brown rice, quinoa, and whole wheat bread over refined grains. Whole grains are rich in fiber and provide sustained energy.

3. Incorporate lean proteins such as chicken, fish, tofu, beans, and legumes. These are important for tissue repair and muscle recovery.

4. Include healthy fats like avocados, nuts, seeds, and olive oil. These fats provide essential fatty acids and help with nutrient absorption.

5. Limit processed foods, sugary drinks, and excessive salt intake. These can negatively impact your health and healing process.

CHAPTER 3

Managing Hormonal Changes

Hormonal changes can occur after a hysterectomy, and certain foods can help support hormonal balance. Here are some foods that may be beneficial:

1. Cruciferous vegetables: Foods like broccoli, cauliflower, kale, and Brussels sprouts contain compounds that support hormone metabolism and balance.

2. Omega-3 fatty acids: Foods rich in omega-3 fatty acids, such as fatty fish (salmon, mackerel,

sardines), flaxseeds, and chia seeds, can help reduce inflammation and support hormonal health.

3. Healthy fats: Including sources of healthy fats like avocados, nuts, seeds, and olive oil in your diet can help support hormone production and balance.

4. Fiber-rich foods: Consuming an adequate amount of fiber from whole grains, fruits, vegetables, and legumes can help regulate hormone levels and support overall digestive health.

5. Phytoestrogen-rich foods: Foods like soybeans, tofu, tempeh, and flaxseeds contain

phytoestrogens, which can help balance hormone levels in the body.

Boosting Energy and Vitality: Recipes for Increased Stamina

Boosting Energy and Vitality: Recipes for Increased Stamina' is your go-to resource for nourishing dishes designed to invigorate body and mind. Packed with nutrient-rich ingredients and tailored to enhance stamina, these recipes will fuel your day, leaving you feeling revitalized and ready to take on any challenge. Elevate your energy levels and embrace a life full of vigor with these delicious, power-packed meals.

To increase stamina for boosting energy and vitality, you can follow these general guidelines:

1. Include nutrient-rich foods: Focus on incorporating foods that are high in vitamins, minerals, and antioxidants. This can include fruits, vegetables, whole grains, lean proteins, and healthy fats.

2. Stay hydrated: Drinking enough water throughout the day is essential for maintaining energy levels. Aim for at least 8 glasses of water per day, and consider adding herbal teas or infused water for added flavor.

3. Prioritize iron-rich foods: Iron is important for energy production, especially for individuals who have undergone a hysterectomy. Include foods like lean meats, beans, lentils, spinach, and

fortified cereals to ensure an adequate intake of iron.

4. Include complex carbohydrates: Complex carbohydrates provide a steady release of energy and can help sustain stamina throughout the day. Opt for whole grains like brown rice, quinoa, oats, and whole wheat bread.

5. Incorporate healthy snacks: Choose snacks that are both satisfying and nutritious. Examples include nuts, seeds, Greek yogurt, fresh fruits, and vegetables with hummus.

6. Consider herbal supplements: Some herbal supplements, such as ginseng or maca root, are

believed to boost energy and vitality. However, it's important to consult with a healthcare professional before incorporating any supplements into your routine.

Supporting Bone Health: Calcium-Rich and Vitamin D-Rich Recipes

In this section, we've curated a selection of delectable recipes designed to fortify your bone health. Packed with calcium-rich ingredients like dairy, leafy greens, and fortified foods, these dishes provide the essential building blocks for strong, resilient bones. From creamy spinach and feta stuffed chicken breasts to a luscious yogurt and berry parfait, each recipe not only delights the palate but also contributes to your overall well-being. Elevate your bone health journey with these nourishing and delicious creations.

1. Include dairy or dairy alternatives: Dairy products like milk, yogurt, and cheese are excellent sources of calcium. If you prefer non-dairy options, consider fortified plant-based milks like almond milk or soy milk.

2. Incorporate leafy greens: Vegetables like kale, spinach, collard greens, and broccoli are rich in calcium. These can be included in salads, stir-fries, or smoothies.

3. Opt for calcium-fortified foods: Look for calcium-fortified foods such as tofu, orange juice, and cereals. These can be a convenient way to increase your calcium intake.

4. Include fatty fish: Fatty fish like salmon, sardines, and mackerel are not only rich in vitamin D but also provide omega-3 fatty acids, which are beneficial for overall health.

5. Get some sunlight: Vitamin D is synthesized in the body when the skin is exposed to sunlight. Aim for 10-15 minutes of sun exposure on your arms and legs a few times a week, preferably during the early morning or late afternoon.

6. Consider supplements: If you're unable to meet your calcium and vitamin D needs through diet alone, your healthcare professional may recommend supplements. It's important to consult with them to determine the appropriate dosage for your specific needs.

Managing Digestive Issues: Recipes for a Healthy Gut

When it comes to managing digestive issues, there are several dietary considerations that can help promote a healthy gut. These include:

1. Fiber-rich foods: Consuming foods high in fiber, such as fruits, vegetables, whole grains, and

legumes, can support healthy digestion and

prevent constipation.

2. Probiotic-rich foods: Probiotics are beneficial

bacteria that can help improve gut health. Foods

like yogurt, kefir, sauerkraut, and kimchi contain

natural probiotics.

3. Hydration: Drinking enough water throughout

the day is essential for maintaining proper

digestion and preventing constipation.

4. Avoiding trigger foods: Certain foods can

exacerbate digestive issues for some individuals.

Common triggers include spicy foods, fatty foods,

caffeine, and alcohol. It's important to identify

and avoid these trigger foods if they affect your digestive system.

As for recipes, these may focus on providing nutritious and easy-to-digest meals for individuals who have undergone a hysterectomy. Some recipe ideas that promote a healthy gut could include:

1. Vegetable stir-fry with tofu or lean protein

2. Quinoa salad with roasted vegetables

3. Baked salmon with steamed asparagus

4. Lentil soup with whole grain bread

5. Smoothies with fruits, leafy greens, and yogurt

CHAPTER 4

Emotional Well-being:Mood-Boosting Foods and Recipes

Emotional well-being is an important aspect of overall health, and certain foods can have a positive impact on mood. Including these mood-boosting foods in your diet can help support emotional well-being:

1. Omega-3 fatty acids: Foods rich in omega-3 fatty acids, such as fatty fish (salmon, mackerel, sardines), walnuts, chia seeds, and flaxseeds, have been linked to improved mood and reduced risk of depression.

2. Complex carbohydrates: Complex carbohydrates, found in whole grains, legumes, and vegetables, can help regulate blood sugar levels and promote the production of serotonin, a neurotransmitter that contributes to feelings of well-being.

3. Foods rich in antioxidants: Antioxidants help reduce inflammation and oxidative stress, which can have a positive impact on mood. Include colorful fruits and vegetables, such as berries, spinach, kale, and bell peppers, in your diet.

4. Probiotic-rich foods: Emerging research suggests a connection between gut health and mood. Consuming probiotic-rich foods, such as

yogurt, kefir, sauerkraut, and kimchi, may help support a healthy gut and potentially improve mood.

 Recipes for a hysterectomy cookbook that focus on emotional well-being, you can consider incorporating these mood-boosting foods into your meals. Here are a few ideas:

1. Grilled salmon with quinoa and roasted vegetables

2. Chickpea curry with brown rice

3. Spinach and berry smoothie with chia seeds

4. Greek yogurt parfait with mixed berries and walnuts

5. Vegetable stir-fry with tofu and brown rice

Maintaining a Healthy Weight: Recipes for Weight Management

Packed with flavorful recipes designed with balance and health in mind, this cookbook makes achieving and sustaining your ideal weight an enjoyable journey. From wholesome breakfast options to satisfying dinners and guilt-free desserts, each recipe is carefully crafted to fuel your body and nourish your soul. With practical tips and a focus on whole, natural ingredients, this book is your key to a vibrant, balanced lifestyle.

1. Focus on balanced meals: Include a variety of fruits, vegetables, whole grains, lean proteins, and

healthy fats in your diet. This will provide essential nutrients while keeping you satisfied.

2. Portion control: Be mindful of portion sizes to avoid overeating. Use smaller plates and bowls, and listen to your body's hunger and fullness cues.

3. Cook at home: Prepare your meals at home as much as possible. This way, you have control over the ingredients and can make healthier choices.

4. Limit processed foods: Processed foods are often high in added sugars, unhealthy fats, and sodium. Opt for whole, unprocessed foods whenever possible.

5. Stay hydrated: Drink plenty of water throughout the day. Sometimes, thirst can be mistaken for hunger, so staying hydrated can help prevent unnecessary snacking.

6. Incorporate physical activity: Regular exercise is crucial for weight management. Find activities you enjoy and make them a part of your routine.

Long-Term Health and Wellness: Recipes for Overall Well-being

Packed with nourishing recipes and expert insights, this book is a blueprint for sustainable well-being. From nutrient-rich meals to mindful eating practices, it offers a holistic approach to health. Embrace a journey towards long-lasting vitality and discover how simple, delicious choices can pave the way for a healthier, happier you.

1. Focus on nutrient-dense foods: Include a variety of fruits, vegetables, whole grains, lean proteins, and healthy fats in your diet. These foods provide essential vitamins, minerals, and antioxidants that support overall health.

2. Prioritize fiber-rich foods: Fiber is important for digestive health and can help prevent constipation, which may be a concern after a

hysterectomy. Include foods like whole grains, legumes, fruits, and vegetables in your meals.

3. Incorporate anti-inflammatory foods: Inflammation can be a concern for some individuals after surgery. Include foods rich in omega-3 fatty acids, such as fatty fish (salmon, mackerel), walnuts, and flaxseeds. Colorful fruits and vegetables, herbs, and spices like turmeric and ginger also have anti-inflammatory properties.

4. Support bone health: Hormonal changes after a hysterectomy can affect bone health. Include calcium-rich foods like dairy products, leafy greens, and fortified plant-based milk alternatives. Vitamin D, which helps with calcium absorption,

can be obtained from sunlight exposure or through dietary sources like fatty fish, egg yolks, and fortified foods.

5. Manage weight: Maintaining a healthy weight is important for overall health. Incorporate the tips I mentioned earlier for weight management, such as balanced meals, portion control, and regular physical activity.

6. Stay hydrated: Drinking enough water is essential for overall health and can help with post-surgery recovery. Aim to drink at least 8 cups (64 ounces) of water per day, or more if recommended by your healthcare professional.

Frequently Asked Questions about Hysterectomy

1. What is a hysterectomy?

A hysterectomy is a surgical procedure in which a woman's uterus is removed. In some cases, other reproductive organs like the ovaries and Fallopian tubes may also be removed.

2. Why is a hysterectomy performed?

Hysterectomies are performed for various medical reasons including conditions like uterine fibroid, endometriosis, gynecologic cancers, chronic pelvic pain, and other serious uterine or pelvic disorders.

3. What are the different types of hysterectomy?

There are different types of hysterectomy surgeries, including total hysterectomy (removal of the uterus and cervix), subtotal or partial hysterectomy (removal of the uterus but leaving the cervix intact), and radical hysterectomy (removal of the uterus, surrounding tissues, and possibly lymph nodes).

4. How is a hysterectomy performed?

A hysterectomy can be performed through various methods including abdominal surgery, vaginal surgery, laparoscopic surgery, or robotic-assisted surgery. The choice of method depends on the patient's specific condition and the surgeon's expertise.

5. Is a hysterectomy reversible?

A hysterectomy is considered a permanent procedure. Once the uterus is removed, it cannot be reattached. It's important for individuals considering a hysterectomy to thoroughly discuss the decision with their healthcare provider.

6. What are the potential risks and complications of a hysterectomy?

While hysterectomy is a common and generally safe procedure, like any surgery, it carries some risks. These may include infection, bleeding, damage to surrounding organs, and anesthesia-related complications.

7. How long is the recovery period after a hysterectomy?

The recovery time can vary depending on the type of hysterectomy and individual factors. Generally, it takes about 4-6 weeks to resume normal activities, but some activities may need to be limited for a longer period.

8. Will a hysterectomy affect hormonal balance?

If the ovaries are also removed during the hysterectomy, it will result in surgical menopause. If the ovaries are left intact, hormonal balance may not be significantly affected.

9. What are alternatives to a hysterectomy?

Depending on the underlying condition, alternatives to hysterectomy may include medication, hormonal therapy, minimally invasive procedures, or conservative surgical approaches.

10. Will a hysterectomy affect sexual function and intimacy?

A hysterectomy can have physical and emotional effects on sexual function. Some women report an improvement in their quality of life and sexual satisfaction after a hysterectomy, while others may experience changes. Open communication with your healthcare provider and partner is essential.

11. How soon after a hysterectomy can I start eating regular meals?

The timing may vary depending on the individual and the type of hysterectomy performed. It is best to consult with your healthcare provider for specific guidance. Generally, a gradual transition to regular meals can begin within a few days to a week after surgery.

12. Are there any dietary restrictions after a hysterectomy?

Again, this can vary depending on the individual and the specific circumstances of the surgery. In general, it is advisable to avoid heavy or greasy foods, as they may be harder to digest during the initial recovery period. It is also important to maintain a balanced diet with plenty of fruits, vegetables, lean proteins, and whole grains to support healing.

13. Can a hysterectomy affect my weight?

Hormonal changes and lifestyle factors can influence weight after a hysterectomy. Some individuals may experience weight gain due to hormonal fluctuations, while others may not notice any significant changes. Maintaining a healthy diet and engaging in regular physical activity can help manage weight and overall well-being.

14. Are there any specific foods that can help with post-hysterectomy recovery?

While there are no specific foods that guarantee a faster recovery, a well-balanced diet rich in nutrients can support healing. Foods high in protein, such as lean meats, fish, beans, and tofu, can aid in tissue repair. Additionally, incorporating foods rich in vitamins A, C, and E, as well as zinc and omega-3 fatty acids, can help support the immune system and reduce inflammation.

Resources and Further Reading

1. "The Hysterectomy Association: Your Hysterectomy Recovery" by Linda Parkinson-Hardman: This book offers practical advice and support for women undergoing hysterectomy, including information on diet and nutrition during recovery.

2. "The Essential Guide to Hysterectomy: Advice from a Gynecologist on Your Choices Before, During, and After Surgery" by Lauren F. Streicher: This comprehensive guide covers various aspects of hysterectomy, including diet

and lifestyle recommendations for optimal recovery.

3. "The Menopause Diet: The Natural Way to Beat Your Symptoms and Lose Weight" by Theresa Cheung: While not specifically focused on hysterectomy, this book provides insights into managing menopause symptoms through diet and nutrition, which can be helpful for women post-hysterectomy.

4. Online resources: Websites such as the American College of Obstetricians and Gynecologists (ACOG) and Mayo Clinic offer reliable information on hysterectomy and post-

surgery care. These websites often have sections

dedicated to diet and nutrition during recovery.

Conclusion

Embracing Your Journey to Health and Healing

As we reach the end of this book, " A Guide to Hysterectomy: Empowering Your Journey to Health and Healing" we want to commend you for your courage, resilience, and commitment to your own well-being. The path you've walked, from considering a hysterectomy to navigating the recovery, is a testament to your strength.

Throughout this book, we aimed to provide not just information, but a hand to hold, and a voice of encouragement. We've covered the practicalities of surgery, the nuances of nutrition, and the complexities of emotions that come with this journey. We've shared stories of strength, and offered insights from experts.

Remember, healing is not just a physical process; it's a holistic endeavor that encompasses mind, body, and spirit. It's about understanding, nurturing, and embracing every facet of your being.

You are not alone in this. You have a support system—family, friends, and healthcare professionals—who stand by you. Your body is capable of remarkable healing, and your spirit, unbreakable.

As you move forward, may you carry with you the knowledge that you have the power to shape your own path to health and happiness. This journey is not just about recovery, but about discovering new strengths within yourself, and emerging even more resilient than before.

You are strong. You are capable. You are worthy of the health and happiness you seek. Your journey continues, and it is one of empowerment, growth, and ultimately, triumph.
With heartfelt wishes for your continued health and healing,

["A Guide to Hysterectomy: Empowering Your Journey to Health and Healing"]

Dr. Rachel Stratford

www.ingramcontent.com/pod-product-compliance
Lightning Source LLC
Chambersburg PA
CBHW050853260726
48660CB00006B/2615